Introduction

I'm going to start this book with [a] suggestion. My suggestion is t[hat you read this book] three times. Read it once throug[h so the infor]mation simply get into your mind. This wil[l allo]w it to become a part of your awareness. Then read it a second time to gain an understanding and perhaps work through the steps. Finally, read it a third time to dive in and get to work, allowing the steps to sink deep in your soul in order to uproot the emotions that are needing to come out.

I've always wanted to write a book. Maybe it's a weird, 'I'll show you stupid teachers and professors!' sort of thing, who knows? There's just something about sharing truths I have learned along the way that is appealing – even compelling. Also, people have often said, "You should write a book." To which I used to reply, "Why? So it can become a doorstop?" because until now the anticipated pain of writing a book has been greater than the anticipated satisfaction at having written a book.

So yes, I have always, secretly, wanted to write a book, lots of books actually. Which is weird because all through high school, and the one semester of community college I attended, I completely sucked at writing. My writing was an epic disaster. In fact, I'm fairly certain that the one semester of English in community college was the catalyst for me to leave college and never return. They said my writing overall was poor, my grammar a travesty and the length of the pieces I wrote, unacceptable. Well, they weren't as eloquent as all that, but you get the idea, right?

I've learned that words can create a self-fulfilling prophecy of sorts. To say my book will be a doorstop would speak its fate as just that. To have the only soul purpose of writing a book be 'make sure it does not end up as a doorstop' is not a huge motivator for writing either. However, when I think of the things I've learned along my journey, far from those community college days, I've realized that I am highly motivated to share those things.

There is a mindset that I have adopted, and my prayer is that it quickly becomes yours as well; if you have an incredible gift, you are morally obligated to share it with the world. Gifts and talents are meant to be shared, not tucked away. If you have an incredible story about rising from the ashes, or a story of recovery and healing, then the same idea applies. You are morally obligated to share it. To tell the world what went down and how you rose again, how you recovered and healed, is your song to sing. And most importantly, you can show others how they could possibly do the same thing, and join in your song.

I have so many dreams and visions, but dealing with my emotional junk, while it has turned into a lovely business journey, seems to have slowed me up a bit more than I would have preferred. So for those of you who would enjoy an emotional roadmap of sorts, through all of your emotional junk, this book is for you!

By the way, many people consume an insane amount of content yet tend to do very little with it. There's the stacks of books on the nightstand, a lengthy rotation of podcasts, a list of saved articles in Facebook to comb through; we consume it all but then what do we do with all of this information?

After you read this book, do something with the information you learned. Don't just chalk it up as another self help, mental health, spiritual awareness book. You're familiar with active listening skills? Read this book using your active reading skills. In fact, if you are not reading this with a journal and pen at your side, stop what you are doing and go get a journal and a pen right now. If you don't have them at your house, get to the Dollar Store or Walgreen's right now – I promise you won't be out more than a few bucks. Take copious notes, underline things, write in the margins. Start this practice now.

Chapter One

begin the begin

Where to start? Do I share with you first about my experiences with getting into this oily business, and my entrepreneur shenanigans? Or should I talk first about my family's literal journey back from the dead and all the attendant emotional baggage claim area trauma from that? If those two stories are separate threads, it's tricky to get them untangled. How about this, let's talk a little about business and personal growth training, because really that combines that topics of business, and emotions.

We have all sat in business training after social media training after personal growth training. All of it is amazing, all of it packed with powerful information… life changing really. Perhaps much of it left you with a feeling of having uncovered what you need to work on, but without the 'how to?' Or maybe you've left, asking, "What do I do with the information I have just received?" Everyone needs a "now what in their life's journey. After spending three years with His followers, Jesus gave His disciples the 'Now what?' "Go into all the world and make disciples of all nations." You need prevention tools. You need practical step by steps.

In every good personal growth or other training you

attend, there is an element of a release that each and every person needs in order to fully walk out the life not that they design, but that life that was designed for them since the foundation of the world. Do you realize that our God has a fairytale life mapped out just for you, since before He knit you together in your mother's womb? He has had a perfect and beautiful plan, just for you.

The challenge is this; most people completely miss it. The enemy of our souls also has a plan of attack, a plan to derail each human on the planet to walk away from the Savior and Creator, and toward his lies and defeat. It's not until much later in life, sadly for some far too late, that we realize this truth, sort of. Even then, sometimes we only half way believe that it's true. We have been so programmed to believe life is hard, challenging, and overwhelming. That oppressed mindset is the paradigm, even though our Jesus said, "I have come to give you life, life in abundance!"

Now, before you come back at me with the verse about Jesus saying that, "in this life we will have trials," allow me to finish the verse for you; "In this life you will have trials, BUT be of good cheer. I have overcome the world." We will discuss that "BUT" much more in a later chapter.

I picture our Savior saying, with a smile on His face, "yes of course, hard times will come, but no worries little one, I got this!" In case you want a full grasp of what overcoming looks like, check out the synonyms for it; defeat, beat, best, conquer, trounce, thrash, rout, vanquish, overwhelm, overpower, destroy, drub, get the better of, triumph over, prevail over, gain a victory over, win over/against, outdo, outclass, outstrip, surpass, excel, worst, subdue, quash, and crush. Jesus has defeated the world, Jesus has conquered the world (yes!), Jesus has overpowered the world, Jesus has outdone the world, Jesus has subdued the world. Jesus has triumphed over the world. Are you getting the point?

So yes, for sure, hard times come. But, we are commanded to *be*; be of good cheer, (cheerful spirits; courage, feasting and merrymaking), because Jesus has overcome.

So we have these thoughts, these patterns, these paradigms that we received from our parents. Many people are so pissed off at their parents because of what they did to them or what crappy parents they were. Listen, stop it. Stop pissing and moaning about how horrible your parents were. I get it, mine were too. But here's a new twist on that old paradigm; have you considered that your parents were doing the best they knew with what had? My mom was abusive. However, she did not know our Jesus and she only did what was within her to do; it was how she was raised and her mom before her. I understand some of you had some heinous situations, so me telling you to stop complaining may likely trigger an emotional response that is unpleasant. Perfect, you're in the right place. You see, once you're finished with this book, you will understand and better grasp how to do just that. When the thought of an unkind parent, sibling, uncle or friend pops in, you will be able to simply say, "they were doing the best they knew how" and move on. Can you imagine what that would look like? Can you imagine the freedom you would feel each day to literally bless and release? Then hang with me fearless reader, we're about to set you free!

The awareness of a need for doing something different is already in you. You picked this book up because in your mind you're thinking, "maybe, just maybe THIS is what catapults me in the right direction!" This is the reason any of us read any of these types of books isn't it? Oh I do pray this is true for you. We are going to dig deep and route out the nonsense that is shackling you to your past. No more will you sit in seminar after seminar writing notes furiously in hopes that you will finally be different, talk different and work different. Once you read through this book and apply the principles inside, you will sit in those same seminars and rather than furiously scribbling every word so you don't forget, you will calmly listen, and write a quote here or there, not so you'll change, but so you will fine tune. Tweak a few things here and there. Perhaps, upgrade to a newer model of your self. By allowing yourself to improve with age, become more beautiful, more poised, and stronger, the confidence you already posses will soar through the roof. Training classes of all kinds will be of greater service to you once you are in the mindset of constantly bettering your mind. You will no longer be looking to find the magic bullet of betterness. You have it right here.

Chapter 2

Where ya goin'?

You have to know where you've been in order to know where you're headed. The challenge is that many people stay stuck in where they've been. They keep looking back, and in doing so steer themselves right off the road. Then they get back on track, look back again, and yep, you guessed it, steer right off the road they were on. It's a cycle, one that gets repeated over and over, after spending thousands on self-improvement and awareness classes.

The key component for anyone looking towards self-improvement is all that stuff between their ears. Oh I know the seminars they are attending speak to this very thing! It's like a mantra - mindset, paradigms, beliefs... But what if you do not know the how? How do you create new beliefs, mindsets and paradigms? If this escapes you, you will forever be on the proverbial hamster wheel of change. How do I know? I know because yours truly was one stuck hamster for evah. I was absolutely one to read book after book, and attend class after class, and yet my brain would betray me. My hamster wheel of choice, the piece from my past that had me mired on the side of the road, was catastrophic expectations. You know about that mindset right? It's the mindset of anticipating the worst possible outcome. Rather than believing for the best, I expected the worst. I would imagine the worst, dream up the worst, and talk about the worst. Then, I would pray against the worst. How sick is that? Jesus says, "do not worry, do not fear, I have overcome", and all of this, yet, here I was, no matter how many notes I took, videos I watched, I assumed the worst.

Even if I didn't go all the way to Technicolor day-dreams of catastrophe, my anticipation was of negative outcomes versus positive. This isn't just a matter of thinking positive or negative. It's more than that. It's literally rewriting your story. Remember cassette tapes? You have a version of that 1980's gem in your mind, telling you the same crappy story over and over. The tapes that are in your head are from personal experience and parent's rhetoric, possibly media influenced. Never mind how they got there, they're just there. And they must be erased and replaced with new tapes, or maybe downloads? Uploads? Whatever the 2019 version would be, do that. That's what needs to happen.

However, we don't ever hear how to accomplish this. We hear, "change your paradigm, change your thinking!" And if you're like me, you're saying to yourself, "Ok! I'll change!" And then, like the saddest trombone sound, you fail miserably and two weeks later, you're back to worst case scenarios.

I mentioned that you have to know where you were before you can move forward. Before you read on, where are you headed? Are you truly in control of your emotions and thoughts or are they in control of you?

Allow me to share a snippet of the harrowing part of our story, the part that shot me into a frenzy of searching for a new mindset, a better way to think, because frankly, I was going off the rails on a crazy train, with no way off.

In the fall of 2010 I received a phone call from a local dermatologist telling me that the mole my son had just had biopsied was a malignant tumor. Zion had melanoma, the deadliest cancer. Our sweet nine year old, pale as anything, the boy who liked to stay inside all the time, had melanoma. From there we radically changed our lifestyle, no sugar, no junk, nothing from a box, removed chemicals from our home and dove into the world of essential oils.

Within about six months we were able to return to a somewhat normal life with routine scans every three to six months, and eventually yearly. A couple of years passed, but we were still living the life of a family that's been marked by pediatric cancer. We hung out with similarly afflicted families, went on a Make A Wish trip to Disney World, and really just talked about cancer all the time. In the midst of that, during a routine ultrasound, we received news that there was something wrong with our fifth child that we were expecting. We learned she would be born with something called omphalocele; all of her organs would be outside her body and she would likely spend six to eight months in the hospital. Even before the cancer we had lost a baby while I was five months pregnant. If you ever doubt the power of a mother's prayer, remember this, the doctor said she would be in the NICU for six to eight months and she was out in thirty days. When she was born the doctors said " oh my gosh! It's not that bad!" Yeah, turns out it was 'only' her liver that was outside her body.

More months went by. Our sweet Selah was home from the hospital, Zion's scans were minimal, at home all was well. All was well, until I started freaking out about things like shoes being in the middle of the floor.... as it turns out, it wasn't about the shoes. I may have been on the verge of a complete breakdown. I had kept life together, still cut hair out of my house to most of the North Dallas suburban moms, home school all but the tiniest of our crew and cooked vegan meals… on a tight budget. Not to mention, every lump and bump that I or the children was intently investigated because surely it was leading to certain death. Once you've been thrown into the world of cancer, it can feel like you're destined for that for the rest of your life. Think about it, how many people do you know that had cancer and then something even worse oame on them. At the time I didn't understand promises I could claim from our God. I didn't really know about not worrying. No one gave me any hope, especially not believers. Most Christians chimed in with "well in this life you will have trials…" Can I tell you something? Do not ever put a period where God puts a comma. Ever. Finish the damn statement, even if you have a hard time believing it. My brain was becoming a giant mind mess. Freak-outs were becoming more common and my anxiety was at an all time high. At one point I checked myself into the ER thinking I was having a heart attack, my chest hurt so bad. Now I understand that to be a panic attack, something many suffer from and take meds for it. What I know now is, panic attacks can be a thing of the past, not a life sentence.

In January of 2015 I was blessed to go to Mona, Utah to visit one of the Young Living farms. While there, some seasoned oilers schooled me on a little friend named Trauma Life. I had no idea oils and emotions were a thing. I was over here trying to diagnose, treat and cure my people. In fact, when my oily friends were buying all these emotional essential oils, secretly I thought they were all a little dramatic and wacko. (Sorry girls! Remember, we don't know what we don't know.) Despite my outright skepticism I went along with it all like a complete weirdo because although I didn't fully believe them, I also didn't not believe them. I bought a truck-load of trauma life, and dutifully applied it to my liver. They told me anger was stored in my liver? Oh boy… little did they know I was rolling my eyes so hard I could see my future and my past. Here's the thing, I had nothing to lose except the few hundred dollars that I had just spent. I used the entire bottle in a month and weirdly enough, I started to see the world differently. My brain started to think differently about situations that would come up. But I had done it wrong. I just slapped on the oil like I got no sense. But it worked. Things in my mind started to change. Not overnight, but I sensed things were a little different. This same miracle bottle went out of stock, and if you use Young Living essential oils, you understand the dire need this puts many of us in. We are at the mercy of our God, rains and weather of all kinds so periodically our beloved oils go out for a time. Trauma Life went out of stock and let me tell you. You want to see a crazy person get crazier? Take away their gateway oil. I scoured the website, books and internet looking for any other oil that would make my brain behave.

Let's pause here; see what happened? The same thing that happens when we sit in classes and self help seminars. We hear the info, apply it, and then go nuts trying to make it stick. Essential oils totally work, but for me, I do not want to replace a drug with a bottle of oil. I want actual physiological change, to not have to strap an oil bottle to my face all day to just get through. These oils have their place, for sure. We must use them daily, as mandated in scripture. However, for true mental health, our God never meant us to be dependent on anything but Him. The essential oils would prove to be a huge value in repairing damaged tissue and replacing negative thought patterns with positive ones. We now use them to keep our bodies strong and as I mentioned, because God set it up since the beginning of time. We use Frankincense during prayer and meditation to create a mindset of what our God thinks.

So I searched. What I realized and would later be able to teach was that all essential oils have an ability to create mental change. Every single one of them.

Chapter 3

The Pursuit of Happiness, but Maybe I Should Not Get My Hopes Up

It was so simple. I was astounded. God had set up millennia ago, at the point of creation, plants to help our brains stay mentally healthy, to have that fairytale life. A fairytale life is nothing more than complete and utter trust in God. Complete trust. Recently I spoke with a woman about life insurance. She said she made her husband get it because after all what if he died?? She and the children would be displaced, she'd have to go to work or they would be destitute!! The amount of crazy coming out of her face was astounding. When I mentioned that God would provide and take care of them, why was she worrying, and wasting money. She said, "well, God let's bad things happen to build character and I just want to be prepared."…

Wow.

There was so very much theologically wrong with that statement. Not wanting to argue with her and create a heated discussion, I dropped it. But it was a profound reminder of that complete lack of trust our culture has created in our faithful so very faithful God. He says, He will NEVER leave you nor forsake you! But we have insurance, life insurance because after all, we have to be prepared in case He chooses to teach us character. Even as I type this, I weep for American Christians. They are missing out on some incredible aspects of God, choosing to look at Him as a stern teacher rather than a kind and loving Father. A perfect Father. Jesus said, "Which of you, if your son asks for bread, will give him a stone? If you, then, though you are evil, know how to give good gifts to your children, how much more will your Father in heaven give good gifts to those who ask him!"

And yet we assume He will give us the stone. So we store up wheat, just in case He chooses to give us that stone or scorpion. We have to make sure we can make our own bread, because we don't remember the scriptures where Jesus fed thousands from a boy's lunch, twice. We forget the story where He makes the beer run at a wedding when it wasn't even His time to start doing miracles.

The problem is not with God. The problem is with you, believing His intent is other than what He so plainly says. The problem was with me, not taking Him at His word when He kept proving Himself over and over, in ways, I don't even know that I can share intelligently. If you want a sneak peek of His miraculous provisions, flipped to end chapter, for story after story about how God showed up in tiny ways and in big ways.

It took just a simple healthy disgust of myself and a lack of belief for me to change. I wish I could say that "oh that one time when He provided a mansion for us to live in", that this was the pivotal point. It wasn't. It was just one day, I was so irritated with myself and made a complete 180. I used the techniques outlined here and did the thing and never looked back. When moments rise up, there are affirmations I can repeat over and over that remind me, He will never leave me nor forsake me. It helps that I have a spirit of being willing to risk everything for the call on my life. If you do not possess this mindset, I suggest you jot that down in your journal. It's powerful.

Maybe you aren't at that stage of healthy disgust with yourself yet. That's okay, you'll get there. You'll get tired of running on whatever your particular hamster wheel is. Where we have dis- ease in our bodies, we will find disease. Do you have dis- ease? Maybe this will spur on the disgust you need in order to change; a Time magazine special showed that happiness, hopefulness, optimism and contentment, appear to reduce the risk or limit the severity of cardiovascular disease, pulmonary disease, diabetes, hypertension, colds and upper-respiratory infections; while depression — the extreme opposite of happiness — can worsen heart disease, diabetes and a host of other illnesses.

Please allow this brief commercial a better way to fuel your body. I'll ask you again, do you have any discomforts? Have any conditions you are currently taking meds for? It's all in your head, literally. I'm going to get in your face for a moment, okay? Do you know God? The Creator of ALL things? Are you currently living with a chronic condition? If so, you'd be an absolute fool to not make a change. He is calling you to this fairytale life and you are living with a condition that is not meant to be your story. Oh I know, God has used your pain as a platform to inspire others. Of course, He wastes nothing, even our foolish years. If you have become emotionally free, changed your diet, and done everything under the sun to create health change and you are still in a chronic state, ok, then I'm wrong, throw this book in the trash. But if you haven't, if you've completely changed to eating plants, but still have mind mess, if you've cleared your mind up, but still eat Chic Fil A, dude, you're doing it wrong.)

Chapter 4

Your Beautiful Brain

From enabling you to think, learn, create, and feel emotions to controlling every blink, breath, and heartbeat—this fantastic switching station is your brain. It is a structure so amazing that a famous scientist once called it "the most complex thing we have yet discovered in our universe". It has been estimated that we have anywhere from 25,000 to 50,000 thoughts a day, and yet we focus on just 10% of those thoughts. Think about that, between 25,000 and 50,000 thoughts each day, yet we are aware of about 2500-5000. Stop for a moment and grasp the last five minutes. Did your mind wander as you read this? Mine did, even as I type. I thought about a post, completely unrelated to this book by the way, that I had seen earlier, which caused an emotional response in me. So even as we are engaged mentally, writing, speaking, or reading, our mind is thinking about other things, in addition to what we are working on.

Now, do this; imagine you are about to jump from an airplane with me. Go ahead, I'll do it too. Your toes are on the edge of the plane, the wind is whipping your face, it's chilly, the instructor is shouting information at you but you can't focus on his words right now~ you're caught up in the moment of the jump, what will it be like? What will it sound like? All of a sudden he shouts, "ONE, TWO, THREE!!! GO

GO GO!"

How do you feel right now, after imagining the jump? You had one of two responses. Either A. you were completely terrified, your palms may have even started to sweat, your heart rate climbed considerably, and your thoughts were racing! Or B. you were completely exhilarated, your palms also may have started to sweat and your heart rate likely also climbed. These are two very different responses to the same situation, yet one we label excitement and one we label terror. In other words your physical feelings and then your emotional response will depend on your thoughts about the situation. Let me explain what I mean.

If you were the one who was excited, you might describe this exercise to someone else as super fun! You were laughing, ready to go sign up for skydiving lessons. If you were on the terror side, you may have thrown this book in the trash and told someone it was a terrible book because it made you think about your worse fear.

Let's do another exercise~

Imagine you have a speech to give, it's an important one, and your friend dares you to stand up, while riding a crowded subway to practice. Would you do it? I'm thinking almost all of you said "no way!" What if I dared you to stand up in front of those people OR jump out of the airplane, now what do you choose?

Thoughts are physical things in your body. They can create physical responses, and cause changes in our bodies. When we have a thought, it creates a feeling. When we have a feeling it creates a hormonal response, releasing that hormone. If there is no feeling there is no hormone; without the hormone there is no feeling. These exercises prove that just by thinking of something terrifying or something exciting, you can create a physical response, thereby creating a hormone release of Adrenaline, Serotonin, cortisol or other hormones that get your blood pumping. Based on what feeling and hormone you release, your body will respond in a fight/flight or freeze mode. A go get it, or a run and hide or stop and do nothing mode.

Understanding our mind and body and the connection between them will help you get to the root of needed support, whether physical or emotional. These are the keys to complete freedom, to move from sitting in all the classes and yet never really grasping the intent, to owning it, changing forever and achieving the greatness you were created for.

Emotions are stored in certain areas in the body. For example; anger and hate are attracted to the liver, grief is stored in the lungs, worry, in the bladder and kidneys. In fact, our emotions can be stored all over. These are just rules of thumb, not hard and fast rules. When our bodies are experiencing negative emotions and these emotions are left unchecked our body will respond by storing these emotions in our tissues.

When there is a reoccurring weakness in the body, this should be a signal to you that there is an emotion trapped in there somewhere. Because all parts of our being interact and work together, if we ignore the role our feelings and thoughts play we are impacting our whole selves. Our body creates a reality based on emotions/thoughts whether they are true or not. Your brain cannot tell the difference between a truth and a lie or fantasy if told over and over. So if you imagined yourself jumping out of an airplane and you felt terrified, then your brain created that physical reaction based on something that wasn't actually happening. If you tell people a lie long enough and hard enough they will eventually believe it. Example- Santa Claus. I rest my case.

Yes, our emotions affect us physically. It might be easy to understand that a scary thought gets our heart beating faster, but it can be harder to realize that loneliness, sadness, or anger can also affect us physically. When it comes to more complex emotions or discomforts few of us consider our emotions to have any relevance. Emotions like hurt, elation, loss, joy, frustration and trust are more complex and seem arbitrary at times. The thing is, all emotions stem from just two emotions, love and fear. That's it. What's cool is knowing and understanding all emotions are so basic, you can then ask yourself "what am I afraid of in this situation? How can I turn the emotion to love?"

Awareness is what gets the ball rolling in the

emotional releasing direction. When a feeling or thought pops in and we start to derail, pause and ask those questions to create awareness.

The only way we can effectively do any of this and understand our emotions and how they affect the body is to understand our brain. We know more about the universe than we do our own brain. We know more about VY Canis Majoris than our own brains. VY Canis Majoris is the largest known star in our universe. Seven quadrillion earths could fit inside VY. That is a 7 with 15 zeros by the way. Who thinks of this stuff? And yet, we know very little about our own brains. We can't change what we don't know about. Our brains our incredibly powerful and capable of so much more, including supporting the body by releasing trapped emotions.

Consider Roger Bannister, remember him? In 1954 he ran the first 4 minute mile. People had said it couldn't be done. Here's the power of our brains, after he did that, scads of other runners were able to run a 4 minute mile. Their brains now knew it was possible. Now, have you heard of James Lawrence? When I heard he completed 50 Ironman races in 50 days I was riveted! I mentioned it to my trainer and he laughed at me and said it couldn't be done and I must have been mistaken. No way. When I met James Lawrence at a Young Living convention 2 years ago, I had PROOF! I heard his testimony. My trainer knew the human body could only take so much of a beating. One Ironman is a 2.2 mile swim, 112 mile bike ride and a marathon, 26.2 miles. In one day. He did that 50 times, oh and in 50 states. When I run, it hurts if I go too far or too fast. My body will wear out. But James Lawrence told his mind, and his mind told his body what to do and it did what it was told. NOT doing it wasn't an option. So his brain followed suit.

When we sit in classes and seminars and trainings on how to do better and be better and goal set and do all the things, we must tap into the emotion of it. The emotional brain is the portion of our brain, our mind really, that will play the biggest part in our sub-conscience, which causes us to move in the world. We call this part of the brain the limbic system. There is a wide range of emotions, including pain, pleasure, docility, affection and anger. The olfactory nerve is connected directly to the limbic system in the brain. This is where approach/avoidance (fight or flight) are created, feelings of being safe or unsafe. The job of the amygdala (part of the limbic system) is to tell us if we are in danger or not. Responses to smells are automatic. Our brains will respond immediately to smells, good and bad. For example, if we smell food that repulses us, it's a survival instinct. We will not be able to eat it. It triggers our amygdala to a fight or flight. If we smell smoke, our bodies will tense up and stop, look around for danger and maybe proceed with caution, or run.

Are you a chronic stress eater? Or are you a snacker? Check this out; the human brain safe guards itself from danger so it tricks you into thinking you're safe because you are eating. So we snack. When animals are in danger they will not eat. But the human brain protects itself by feeding the body, which leaves it feeling more safe. See how that works? So the next time you snack or stress eat, rather than judging yourself and becoming angry, be kind to yourself. Understand that you may be in a space that requires extra grounding. Our brains are simply remarkable. But do you really understand the science behind it?

The fact that you need comfort means you feel unsafe. What's going on that you feel scared? Unsafe? Triggered?

Rather than chastise ourselves for snacking in the wee hours, why not recognize that you just might feel "a way" and have a need to ground and create the illusion of safety?

If you feel triggered, be aware.
Don't beat yourself up.
Recognize that you feel like you are needing a blanket of feel good food.

Chapter 5

Speaking Life

Learning how the brain works is important, and what you do with that information will be the turning point for you and your emotional growth. You can choose to let the knowledge that your thoughts control your actions roll around in your mind, thinking, 'that's nice. I wonder if that would help me?" And perhaps you move on with your life. Or, you can draw a line in the sand, today, not tomorrow, but today and change.

If you're inclined to do that latter, then stop everything. Grab a journal, a notebook, something to write in. Do not read past this point without your journal. If you do, you will likely be like countless thousands who hear this information and give a nod to it, but sadly do not put it into action. This is what is missing from every class, every workshop and seminar you have sat in. Make the change, today.

The first change to our brains that we must make is the story we tell ourselves. You can call it speaking life, or truth or affirmations. My preference is "affirmations". If you are over the age of 45, like me, you remember the SNL sketch, Stuart Smalley, when he looks in a mirror and says "I'm good enough, I'm smart enough, and doggone it, people like me!" This is probably the picture in your mind when you hear the word affirmations. In satirical fashion, this skit made us laugh at people who use affirmations. The truth is, affirmations are critical to changing the brain. Scripture says in Philippians 4:8, "Finally, brothers and sisters, whatever is true, whatever is noble, whatever is right, whatever is pure, whatever is lovely, whatever is admirable—if anything is excellent or praiseworthy—think about such things." In addition, Romans 12:2 says, "Do not conform to the pattern of this world, but be transformed by the renewing of your mind. Then you will be able to test and approve what God's will is—his good, pleasing and perfect will". They work. They are vital to our emotional well being.

Be transformed by the renewing of your mind... how can you renew it, then be transformed if you tell yourself the same nonsense you've always told yourself. It has to change, it must be audible and it must be different.

The root word for affirmation is the Latin word, Affirmare which means to STRENGTHEN, to MAKE STEADY. What lifting weights will do for our muscles, affirmations will do for our brain! With every word we speak over ourselves, we strengthen that mental muscle more each day. Affirmations are a form of autosuggestion. When practiced deliberately and repeatedly they reinforce chemical pathways in the brain, strengthening neural connections. They enforce those neurons that fire together and grow new pathways, making it easier for our brain to continue on a positive path toward our goals and intentions. Affirmations detox our thoughts and restructure the dynamic of our brains so that we begin to think in the way we were designed. When we verbally affirm our dreams, desired emotions and ambitions, we are instantly empowered with a deep sense of reassurance that our wishful words become reality. Saying these words to ourselves creates a reality of who we actually are. We see ourselves how our Creator sees us. Often times, we see ourselves through the eyes of our circumstances, rather than who we are. Someone once said, 'where you are is not who you are.' Wise words.

We are not the sum total of our circumstances.

We are not the abuse we encountered.

We are not the job we are in.

We are not the position we hold.

We are created in the image of an amazing and loving God. We are His child, no more no less. In Christ~

We are perfect.

We are worthy.

We are royalty.

We are chosen.

We are loved.

This is your reality if you are in Christ. It's beautiful. More than that, with this knowledge in mind, I cannot fathom why anyone would think it odd to speak powerful words over themselves, it's more odd that we aren't all wearing signs saying each one of these things, encouraging life wherever we go!

No matter what your current reality is, speaking words that align with your desire for emotional freedom will propel you toward that freedom and bring about lasting change. Then and only then will you move into the reality you are wanting.

If you are accustomed to using essential oils, then at this point take out your Cedar wood. If you do not currently use essential oils, do not be concerned. Also, do not go to the local market and purchase any old essential oil. Not all essential oils are created equal. Because this is not a book about which essential oil company is the best, I will not take up an entire section describing Seed to Seal, or farms. What I will say is this; you trusted me enough to purchase this book, you trusted me enough to go this far in he book, will you trust me when I say, only Young Living essential oils will do for you? You are better than cheap imitations.

These steps can all be practiced without the help of essential oils, however, the process goes a hell of a lot faster and they last much longer. It's your choice.

At this point Cedar wood is the essential oil of choice. Oh and PS- you're not allergic to cedar wood essential oil, especially if it is the species Cedrus Atlantica. Again, not an essential oil book, but I can hear some of your thoughts. It's virtually impossible to be allergic to TRUE essential oils, something about proteins, aminos etc. Look it up, education is power.

If you have heard me speak, then this recommendation would come as no surprise. But why am I always saying Cedar wood first? First of all you need to understand how essential oils work in the brain. Fragrance is the substance of memories. Research shows that when inhaling essential oils, it can stimulate the olfactory receptors and activate regions in the brain's limbic system associated with memory, emotion, and state of mind. This is the brain's center of emotion and memory as well as the "unconscious brain." In less than a second, a scent has the power to trigger a number of physical and emotional responses that, perhaps, you have long forgotten about.

Also, essential oils work by calming the central nervous system and helping us to relax instead of allowing the buildup of stress in the body. Essential oils can help in the release of old emotional hurts. In 1989, Dr Joseph Ledoux from NY Medical University discovered that the amygdala (in the limbic center of the brain) plays a role in the storage and release of emotional hurts. He also suggested that aromas could trigger an emotional release. As mentioned earlier, our sense of smell activates the limbic system. Finally, and this is where Cedar wood comes in, essential oils carry molecules known as sesquiterpenes, which are capable of penetrating the bloodbrain barrier. Cedar wood has the highest concentration of sesquiterpenes, higher than any other essential oil. This powerhouse oil removes emotional blockers that hinder you to learn. At minimum, you should have a bottle of Cedar wood at the ready.

If I were to ask you, "why are you reading this book?" likely you'd tell me, freedom. You are in search of emotional freedom, and maybe, just maybe this will be the answer. Oh I pray so, my friend. The very thing that keeps us from being truly free is FEAR. We mentioned before, but I'll say it louder for those in the back. ALL negative emotions stem from this one emotion, FEAR. Let's kick fear to the curb, once and for ALL!

First of all know this, and commit it to memory; for God has not given us the spirit of fear; but of power, and of love, and of a sound mind. That's found in 2 Timothy 1:7. If you know God, then you have a spirit of LOVE, of POWER, and of a SOUND MIND. You already have that.

Take your Cedar wood, drip 2-3 drops in the palm of your hand and inhale with a deep belly breath. The kind that makes your belly stick way out. Breathe deep, from the bottom of your gut, for a count of four. Now exhaled for that same count of four. Now write in your journal for at least five minutes. Set a timer if you need, and write everything you would like to believe is true of you. Borrow my belief in you if you need a greater supply. Below are several affirmations that I have written, please utilize them as your own if believing truth about yourself is challenging at this point. Be sure your affirmation is set in the present tense, "I am ____, I have ____, I choose___".

Add cedar wood essential oil to your diffuser throughout the day and as you walk by the diffuser, think on these truths that you are writing.

Affirmations

"I am loved."

"I am special."

"I am a child of God."

"I am priceless."

"I am richly blessed in all ways."

"I create meaningful relationships."

"I create an extraordinary life."

"I make space for harmony."

"I make space for abundance."

"I am calm."

"I am peaceful in all situations."

"I have a spirit of power, love and a sound mind."

"I am contagious peace."

"I am free."

Chapter 6

Emotions in the Body

This is a huge topic. There is much research now on the fact that emotions are not only stored in the body, but that these same negative emotions can make us sick. Emotions are big, friends.

- Let's repeat that. Emotions are big.
- Feelings are big.
- Feelings are important.
- Emotions are important.

This is the key thing to remind ourselves of, especially when we are speaking to our children. In our house we learned the hard way that categorizing feelings as small, medium and large did not create freedom for our children. It created hurt and resentment. No matter what you are feeling, it needs to be addressed, and not told it is silly or dumb or worst, unimportant.

Here is a list, though not exhaustive, of our organs and the emotions that can become trapped along with the reoccurring weakness.

Right shoulder- outer world burdens

Left shoulder- inner world burdens

Throat center- self-expression issue, lack of trust, inability to speak feelings. This one in particular I find interesting, since many women have thyroid challenges. This is not a coincidence.

Heart center- grief, sorrow, sadness and loss. Emptiness of heart, lack of love. helplessness, aloneness, disillusionment, embarrassment, shame, humiliation, repressed feelings, disappointment, genetic memory, cruelty or meanness.

Liver - anger and rage, anger at others, anger at self, jealousy, resentment.

Gut- fear and phobias, loss of control, fear of losing control, giving our power to another person, and relationships.

Pelvic and Reproductive area- family sexual issues, childhood conditioning, survival, feeling we won't survive a life-threatening incident. Violations related to surviving (abuse, violence, rape, accidents). Can result in impotence and frigidity.

Spleen- guilt, unacceptance, self judgment, self criticism, not deserving of good life as for us, inability to accept and receive.

Left Hip-lack of emotional support

Right hip- lack of financial support.

When we have reoccurring weakness, 99% of the time it's a manifestation of emotional struggles. The condition however, may not result for years after the event. This is why it is so important to keep clearing those emotions and emotional trauma.

I mentioned in the previous chapter, we have about 25,000-50,000 thoughts per day, and focus on very few of them. Thoughts create physical responses in the body. Here's where we need to be mindful of every feeling we have, and not stuff them down; when our bodies experience tough emotions and they are left unchecked/not dealt with, our body will respond by storing these emotions in our organs. In addition, our brain will create a "file" and store the emotion and thought pattern to go with it in the file in order to keep us safe. We are wired for survival. Our brain is quite busy, and extremely efficient. It needs to keep it moving in order to keep us alive. For example, if a child experiences a traumatic event, many times the brain will store that memory so deep, as the child grows, that event may not be in the fore front of their mind, they may experience gaps in their memory surrounding other less traumatic events. Abuse victims can be accused of lying, simply because they cannot remember specific details. The truth is, their brain allowed not only that memory to be fuzzy, but other memories during that time to be hard to recall.

Do you or your children have a reoccurring weakness or issue? Write the condition in your journal. This is where essential oils are powerful for releasing trapped trauma. They give the brain a safe space to release and allow healing to begin in the body where the emotion was stored. Trauma Life, in my opinion, is the best essential oil blend to start the process of release. It's incredibly gentle and not over powering as far as scents go.

Here's the process: add 1-3 drops in your palms and breathe into the specific space in your body where you feel the weakness. Do you know what I mean when I say breathe into it? It's a matter of focusing on the space and imagining clean, pure, fresh oxygen flowing into that area as you breathe in for a count of four. As you exhale, imagine the pain and weakness leaving that space. Sometimes placing one hand on the area and the other hand cupped over your nose as you deep breathe, will allow the body to respond as the mind reacts to the scent.

The word "aromatherapy" is derived from the Latin word *aroma*, and the French word *thérapie*. Here's a little history for those of you not currently using essential oils. In the 1920's, a French chemist and perfumer by the name of René-Maurice Gattefossé became interested in the use of essential oils for their medicinal properties after he burned his arm. He applied lavender essential oil and put it on the burn to discover it healed quickly and no scar was left. This event led to his ongoing study of the use of essential oils for medicinal purposes. It is Gattefossé that is credited with coining the term *aromatherapy* in 1928. Gattefossé wrote a book called *Aromathérapie: Les Huiles essentielles hormones végétales* that was later translated into English and named Gattefossé's Aromatherapy.

I feel at this point it's important to share some science with you about how essential oils work in the body and the chemistry behind them. Once you grasp this, the physical changes they make, that I'm talking about here, will be more believable. One drop of essential oil contains approximately 40 million-trillion molecules. Numerically that is a 4 with 19 zeros after it: 40,000,000,000,000,000,000. We have a mere 100 trillion cells in our bodies. So just one drop of essential oil contains enough molecules to cover every cell in our bodies with 40,000 molecules. Considering it only takes one molecule of the right kind to open a receptor site and communicate with the DNA to alter cellular function, you can see why even inhaling a small amount of oil vapor can have profound effects on the body, brain, and emotions. Research shows that when inhaling the constituents in essential oils, it can stimulate the olfactory receptors and activate regions in the brain's limbic system associated with memory, emotion, and state of mind. This is the brain's center of emotion and memory as well as the "subconscious brain." In less than a second, a scent has the power to activate a number of physical and emotional responses that, perhaps, you have long forgotten about or believed were not an issue any more.

Certain essential oils work by calming the central nervous system and helping us to relax instead of allowing the buildup of anxiousness in the body.

The amygdala is the "watchdog" of the brain. It is constantly looking to identify "friend" or "foe" in our environments. In a matter of seconds, we can be triggered into a fight/ flight/freeze response and locked in the "downstairs brain" unable to access our "upstairs" or the executive (logic and reason) brain. If we stay in the locked down state - in the downstairs survival brain for too long, our brain will begin to rewire itself. Our body will actually carve pathways in our brain, suppressing our emotions and the ability to attach and connect to others.

Conversely, as we start to release these trapped emotions, we can rewire the brain with new pathways, allowing our brains and ultimately our bodies to thrive!

Know your oils and what makes them powerful;

- **Phenols** are the constituents in essential oils that are stimulating to the nervous and immune systems. They clean and purify the receptor sites of cells. They have antioxidant properties and a high level of oxygenating molecules. Without clean receptor sites, cells cannot communicate, and the body malfunctions resulting in sickness. This graphic is a simple visual of the phenols job.

- **Sesquiterpenes**- After the phenols finish their work, sesquiterpenes are up to bat. These constituents erase miswritten information in your DNA. They are present in almost all essential oils. The chemistry of essential oils tells us that they are the largest group of terpenes known naturally in the plant and animal kingdom! They are larger than monoterpenes and are very viscous (stickier consistency) so they are often used as fixatives in the perfume industry.

- **Monoterpenes**- Last and certainly not least, the monoterpenes are up for their job. These powerhouse constituents seek to repair any damage to the cells. Think about your cell phone, sometimes it just needs to return to basic settings in order for the new programs to be installed. Notice that Frankincense is a monoterpene intense essential oil. Also notice that Frankincense is in almost every emotional blend that Gary Young created.

As you work through this process, choosing the essential oils that are best for you, particularly when we discuss triggers is very individual. Go to your favorite oils, the ones you would love to crawl in the bottle with if you could. What is their highest constituent? Are they higher in sesquiterpenes or monoterpenes? Add these to your emotional releasing arsenal. There is a reason you were attracted to those oils. Give careful thought to the new program you desire to rewrite in your brain.

Journal the new thought patterns you are choosing to write in your brain, tonight before you sleep. Apply your favorite essential oils as you do this. Journaling things for which you are grateful in the evening is a powerful way to keep your brain rewiring into a positive mindset. As you sleep, your brain works out the day, so if the last thing you thought was something you were grateful for, your mind will start engaging in all kinds of happiness and joy throughout the day. Once you have written, close your eyes, breathe the oils in again, and imagine each molecule erasing old negative pathways, resetting your brain, entering in new programs, healthy, strong, and powerful thoughts. Imagine your brain growing and feeling stronger with each breath. If you're one to remember your dreams, write down what you dreamt tomorrow morning. When we journal and use oils at night, our brains work out and release what we need to while we sleep, many times the form of dreams. It's powerful!

Let's talk about identifying emotions. As I have mentioned, all emotions stem from two basic ones, love and fear. Knowing that positive emotions are based in love and negative emotions are based in fear will create a simpler categorization for you as you process these. Remember to ask yourself these questions; What am I afraid of? Who am I afraid of?

What is it I am loving? Who am I loving? Why it is, at times, hard to believe positive things about yourself?

Have you wrestled with the affirmation portion of this book? How easy has it been for you to continue to speak life over yourself in the form of affirmations so far? If you have been telling yourself a story based in fear then your brain will be grappling with these new concepts you're feeding it. Maybe it's not even your fear, maybe it's someone else's that they spoke over you. No matter, it's time to route it out.

The body creates a reality based on these emotions/ thoughts, whether they are true or not. Our brain cannot tell the difference between a truth and a lie if told over and over. If you tell people a lie long enough and hard enough they will eventually believe it. As you say your affirmations, let me encourage you to stand firm as the scripture says, and say them a little louder today. There are commands in Scripture that are repeated many times. The call to 'stand firm' is one of those commands. It appears all throughout the Bible.

In case you need a reminder, here are seven powerful verses in Scripture about standing firm:

Ephesians 6:11
"Put on the full armor of God, so that you will be able to stand firm against the schemes of the devil."

Ephesians 6:13

"Therefore put on the full armor of God, so that when the day of evil comes, you may be able to stand your ground, and after you have done everything, to stand."

1 Peter 5:9

"But resist him, firm in your faith, knowing that the same experiences of suffering are being accomplished by your brethren who are in the world."

1 Corinthians 15:58

"Be steadfast, immovable, always abounding in the work of the Lord."

Philippians 1:27

"Conduct yourselves in a manner worthy of the gospel of Christ, so that whether I come and see you or remain absent, I will hear of you that you are standing firm in one spirit, with one mind striving together for the faith of the gospel."

1 Corinthians 16:13

"Be on the alert, stand firm in the faith, act like men, be strong."

Philippians 4:1

"Therefore, my beloved brethren whom I long to see, my joy and crown, in this way stand firm in the Lord, my beloved."

This verse, 1 Corithians 15 gets me every time. Be immovable, steadfast. I picture a mountain or an anchored ship. Anchored on every side. Do you feel immovable, and steadfast in all things? It's time to say those affirmations with a lot more force. Say them seven times. Say them in different ways. Get your brain completely engaged and on board with your new thought patterns. Soon these thoughts will be really rooted in your neuro pathways. Most of all, be loving to yourself. If thoughts of doubt creep in, acknowledge them, but let it pass. Don't judge it. Understand this is a process that takes practice. Practice often throughout each day and trust the process.

Fear is sneaky. What is in your environment, that you can control, that may be causing you to have fear as part of your mind? Is it time to evaluate your circle of friendships? Is your social media newsfeed overly riddled with fear posts and hype? I've quoted this scripture already, and I'll keep quoting it until you have it so imbedded in your mind that you'll say it before I have even typed it out. "Whatever is true, whatever is lovely, whatever is good, whatever is honorable, whatever is right, if there is any excellence and if anything is worthy of praise, dwell on these things." You do realize don't you that the words in our scripture are for a life giving purpose? It's not a list of rules, or dos and don'ts. They are for life and godliness, to keep you safe, healthy and strong.

Is your mind filled with these things? What is within your control to have this be true of you? Are there groups you need to step away from? How can you audit your surroundings to create a more life giving and peaceful environment?
Some situations may be beyond your control, where there are less than lovely situations. Yet what is in your power to add in is positive thoughts, positive music, and positive friendships. Even when we have situations and people we must see often, that might threaten our mindset or peace, we can control how we respond. We can imagine ourselves into a better frame of mind before the situation arises. We'll spend some time in the next chapter discussing triggers and some anti-trigger tactics.

Chapter 7

Triggers

Up until now we've been shaking off the cobwebs of your emotional brain, and your limbic system. The information shared so far has increased your awareness of some simple basics of your emotions, feelings and your responses to them. Image you decided to start lifting weights. The first few weeks of physical training is a matter of understanding the weights, the machines and what your body can reasonably withstand. Or for my readers who run, the first time you ever started running was simpler than weight lifting, yet no different in the necessity of understanding the mechanics of it. In fact, running might be a better metaphor here because in order to run well, you must understand and fully appreciate your body and how it works. In running, you wouldn't stay at the same pace if you kept running over a period of weeks, months, and years. If fact, your body would push you further and/or faster. Same with weight training, your trainer would start to push you toward heavier weights and toward exercises that were more complex in terms of the amount of different muscles involved. In both cases, you're getting stronger, faster and overall healthier than before.

As you continue on this journey of freedom, it may start to hurt, as would weight training or running. If the journey starts to get a little heavier and you feel as if you want to stop, take a breath, and slow down, but don't stop. Imagine what you might possibly throw away if you give up. Imagine all that you'll gain if you press on.

Before you read on, take a drop each Frankincense, Stress Away and Lavender essential oils, activate them in your hand by rubbing your hands clockwise, make a little tent with your hands over your nose and breathe them in. Take a deep breath and count, 1, 2, 3,4 and then blow it out 1,2,3,4. Let's do this for a total of five times. Each time, notice how your belly sticks out as you inhale. This is by design. Filling our diaphragm with fresh oxygenated air brings so much life! We will continue to practice breathing throughout the duration of this book. For now remember this; breathing is key to releasing emotions, and heading triggers off at the pass.

Triggers are a huge deal and must be understood in order to completely be free. A trigger is something that sets off a memory tape or flashback transporting the person back to the event of her/his original trauma. Triggers are very personal; different things trigger different people. A person's triggers are activated through one or more of the five senses: sight, sound, touch, smell and taste. We all have emotional triggers. That feeling when someone makes a jokingly-mean comment that might not be a huge deal to another person, but completely takes you out emotionally for the rest of the day? You may find yourself feeling off center and feeling emotions that don't seem to match your current situation.

Side note to a child, having to give up a favorite toy for a sibling to play with is, in their minds, traumatic. Remember on day 2 we said emotions are big? Do not judge whether your experience is "true" trauma. If you're triggered, your mind/body feel there was trauma. Acknowledge it and give scores of grace. It can be challenging to identify what exactly our triggers are, but this process of getting to know and understand them can help us heal, and learn how to thrive.

Why do we all have triggers? Simply put, we were all children once. When we were growing up, we inevitably experienced pain or suffering that we could not acknowledge or were not allowed to deal with appropriately at the time. As adults, we become triggered by experiences that are reminiscent of these old painful feelings. Many times people will turn to a habitual or addictive way of trying to manage the painful feelings, i.e. overeating, overworking, over whatever brings instant pleasure to squash the triggered painful emotion. Think about some ways that you might be triggered on a daily basis. Pause when you feel an emotional response rise up that seems "overly emotional". Take a moment to ask yourself, "Why am I being triggered by this?" If your brain allows you to find the answer, write that down.

And then grab your Trauma Life and apply it over your liver, your shoulders and any where else you feel tension as a result of the trigger. If you are in a place to journal, write the feeling that goes along with it, where do you feel the trigger? How do you see the world now? Is it hard? Do you struggle with accomplishing your task after being triggered? Write out the truth of what's happening now, versus what happened that created the trauma. It's important to look for the truth if you get triggered; this is our way out response. It's the way we will stop the trigger in its tracks and respond appropriately.

If these steps are difficult, take them slow. One at a time even. Be sure to keep applying the oils as you transition to the next step.

Now that you are fully aware of what triggers you, it's time to learn how to head them off at the pass. In a perfect world we would never be triggered again. People are still people and we are responsible for how we react to them or a given situation.

This is being emotionally of sound mind. If we allow ourselves to be ruled by the triggers, we are not of an emotionally sound mind. In fact we tend to act like crazy people, having a total out of body experience. As mentioned, the triggers may cause us to respond in ways that do not match the circumstance. Being emotionally sound means we don't stuff the feelings and emotions, rather, we acknowledge it, and understand fully what is happening, but rather than letting it fully consume us, we pause and deal appropriately with them.

Being emotionally sound starts with breathing. Did you know most people breathe incorrectly? We tend to take shallow, more hurried breaths, especially when triggered. This is a survival skill that we must have. Taking short breaths in order to start a full on sprint is key for survival.
However, when we are triggered and an emotion arises, we should not take short breaths, because there is no real need to start running. Our brain is telling us to take flight, but that is unnecessary. Taking slow, deep, and long breaths create space in our lungs and belly so that the trapped emotions can be released.

As you read through this next portion, take the HIGHEST frequency oil you can find and apply it on your chest, over your heart and on your forehead. At this point I suspect you have chosen to use essential oils for this freedom process. If you do not have essential oils yet, that is okay. As I mentioned, you can become emotionally sound without them, but why you'd want to do this process without them, I have no idea. So if you have chosen to walk this path without essential oils, then be sure to turn on some high frequency music, brew high frequency tea (no microwaves please), or eat a bit of high frequency foods like dark berries and fair trade chocolate.

Chapter 8

Steps to release triggers

Step one:

Practice deep breaths and also as you breathe, create awareness of where you want that breath to go. Where in your body are you feeling triggered? Breathe into that space. Have you ever noticed that when you get nervous, say before a presentation or before a big discussion, you start to have physical responses? Maybe you then talk fast, you move your hands a lot. Slow down. Breathe.

Step Two:

Ground yourself. Remember, scripture is clear, STAND FIRM it says. Go back to the last chapter and reread the verse about standing firm. Stand your ground, be immovable, and unshakable. Grounding ourselves is the act of standing firm. We can ground by either applying grounding oils, tree oils for example, or ground by taking your shoes off and letting your feet be on the earth, or my favorite, both. As you breathe, stand firm. Stand up if needed, placing your hands on your hips to stabilize yourself. Feel the power of the ground firmly planted beneath both your feet. Grounding is an exercise that connects you energetically to the earth. It allows you to be more in the present moment, and to receive nourishing energy.

Do you snack when you are stressed? Your body is asking for more grounding. Don't be harsh with yourself, acknowledge the need to ground and make the choice to care for yourself with a grounding exercise before you grab a snack.
Not being grounded creates the feeling of being unfocused, easily distracted, in chaos, missing in action, anxious, powerless and unsafe. It increases the chances of those triggers staying with you. Being ungrounded can make you feel like you are out of control and tossed around by every circumstance that comes along, because you are easily influenced by your environment and other people's feelings.

Step Three:

Practice being intentional with not just words, but with your emotional intelligence as well. How do you respond in a triggering situation and then how would you like to respond? What response makes you feel the most empowered? Practice the intention you have along with the outcome you desire in every situation. Now you are able to create the future reality you desire by practicing with a purpose. You know what you want, and you now have the tools to get it. Imagine being in complete control of your responses. Imagine how incredible it will feel to be in control of your emotions and responses. Practice daily in a space where you are not being triggered. Remember, first responders and military personal do not prepare for emergencies and wars during emergencies and wartime. They have drills. They practice. Go and do likewise.

Essential oil users, carry your anti-trigger oils 24/7. This is why you'll hear people who utilize the power of essential oils mention they will not ever leave home without their oils. It's a way of staying emotionally free. You never know when something will pop up, so be prepared.

Chapter 9

PTSD

After learning about and identifying triggers, it's time to open up the PTSD conversation.

What is Post Traumatic Stress Disorder? PTSD is a condition of persistent mental and emotional stress occurring as a result of injury or severe psychological shock, typically creating a disturbance of sleep and a constant vivid recall of the experience.

PTSD comes in all shapes and sizes. Before you blow this chapter off, thinking your emotional struggle does not fall under PTSD, remember, your brain perceives circumstances how it perceives it. You actually do not get to choose whether you have PTSD or trauma, or whether you do not. Your brain decides. So stop categorizing what is "true trauma" and ask your brain and body, 'is this something I should be aware of?'

There is no need to judge it, only to recognize the responses you have and respond appropriately so you can heal and move forward. Unfortunately we live in a culture where the law of relativity reigns supreme. Everything is relative. We compare and contrast, ie "this person has it way worse", or, "well at least I have xyz still."

Thanks to White Christmas and the Christian culture in the U.S., we have been told to count our blessings. True, scripture does say, 'count it all joy when you fall into various trials'. What it does not say is sweep under the rug the trauma and hardships you've endured. Scripture also encourages us to comfort each other with the comfort we have received in the midst of our own hardships. Mourn with those who mourn, rejoice with those who rejoice. It's both/and. In the west, we have this terrible habit of comparing and contrasting circumstances. We judge hardships. Listen, hard is hard. If your stuff feels hard, then it is your hard. My stuff may not appear as challenging to you, but that's none of your business. It's hard to me. Your stuff may seem simple and bearable to me, yet again, it's none of my damn business. It's your hard, not mine. Scripture does not tell us to judge someone's burden and tell them they should count their blessings. In fact, can we just stop that nonsense, please? Rather, can we seek to understand one another, seek to pursue peace and rather than tell someone to count their blessings, actually become a blessing for others? What a beautiful vision our Christian culture would be if we followed what scripture said, to the letter. Love, peace, understanding.

Still not convinced that you or your loved one falls into the PTSD category?

Check out these three characteristics to see if this resonates:

1)Re-experiencing the trauma through intrusive distressing recollections of the event, flashbacks, and nightmares.

2) Emotional numbness and avoidance of places, people, and activities that are reminders of the trauma.
side note many people consider themselves introverts because they avoid people, but in actuality they are experiencing some form of residual trauma that makes them uncomfortable around others.

3) Increased arousal such as difficulty sleeping and concentrating, feeling jumpy, and being easily irritated and angered.

Here are some ways trauma manifests in individuals:

1) Inability to remember an important aspect of the traumatic events. You know how abused women are accused of not being able to remember details? It doesn't mean they are lying, it means their brain was protecting them. Please don't ever accuse a woman of lying again, it's none of your damn business. Always, always believe a woman who says she's been abused. Always.

2) Persistent and exaggerated negative beliefs or

expectations about themselves, others, or the world (i.e., "I am bad," "No one can be trusted," "The world is completely dangerous").

3) Persistent and/or distorted blame of self or others about the cause or consequences of the traumatic events.

4) Persistent fear, horror, anger, guilt, or shame.

5) Diminished interest or participation in significant activities.

6) Feelings of detachment or estrangement from others.

7) Persistent inability to experience positive emotions.

This is not an exhaustive list, it's just a grouping of major manifestations.

In emotional healing there is no magic bullet for folks experiencing distress. Pairing essential oils with emotional releasing is not a one size fits all. In fact, some oils can be a trigger because of the type of trauma someone has experienced. For example, lavender was an oil that set me on edge on my first go round of using it. I powered through because that is what was taught to me. Lavender is an oil that is specific to releasing abandonment issues. It was doing it's work on me and I was simply not ready. However, an oil like Frankincense I found warm and soothing. Best practice is to start with the essential oil that brings peace of mind and joy when first inhaled. That's when you know you've found your magic bullet. If you have concerns about possibly being triggered, start slow. Use your essential oils in a diffuser only, do not apply topically until you are sure the oil is a delight to you.

If you have found yourself in the PTSD category and you think, oh super, now what? Do not worry, I won't leave you hanging. For now, as you continue along use your Valor and Trauma Life.

Please understand that everything I share in this book, I myself have walked through, and have walked others through it with great success. If you feel ready to tackle your PTSD follow these next steps. Do not do this portion if you are just learning about trauma and the affects of it. Again, take it slow. Go back to the previous chapter and work through that section again. Become comfortable with the uncomfortable.

Next steps:

1. Write your traumatized self a letter of apology for forcing her/him to rationalize the event, for not supporting her/him in a way that that younger person needed. Trust me, this one step will bring so much

healing.

2. Apply your Forgiveness for this next step. Write a letter of forgiveness to your now self. Many of us needed to just forgive ourselves before we can find complete healing. Before we can even think of forgiving someone else, forgiving ourselves is critical. Many people rush to forgiving someone else because it is mandated in scripture. True yes, and I believe our Jesus would completely be fine with us starting the forgiveness process with ourselves first. In fact, He doesn't care who you forgive first, it's that you actually do forgive that is important.

If you realize that your child may be struggling with some sort of trauma, have a conversation. Sometimes children don't know that it is acceptable to share. Be sure you are not sitting face to face with your child. It can be a trigger, particularly if your child sits on the Autism or Aspergers spectrum. Respect their boundaries as you would have wanted someone to respect yours. Take them out on a walk, and be sure you share with them you are going to have a talk like this. Apply Valor on them as well, and for sure White Angelica on yourself.

Chapter 10

Growth From Trauma

Identifying PTSD is one thing, healing from it is a whole other ballgame. This is where growth from trauma comes in. Rather than focus on post traumatic stress, we now can turn our attention to growing from trauma, and even thriving as a result of the trauma. This takes work, a lot of work, and it is possible. It is possible to turn the pain into joy, the mourning into dancing. If it wasn't possible, scripture would not speak to that. Jesus came so that we could be set free from our pain. He uses these traumas and trials in order to bring freedom in our lives and well as others.

Growing from trauma can be a positive change experienced as a result of the struggle with a major life crisis or a traumatic event. How we go about growing from trauma is as individual as our essential oils themselves.

First, we must recognize that the whole-person healing includes physical, mental, emotional, spiritual and social wellness. Of course there are even more ways to use our essential oils therapeutically, but these will be a jumping point.

As you recover and find growth from trauma, you may additionally find spiritual needs that were not previously recognized. Frankincense essential oil will create a mental environment that will assist you in reconnecting with God. It's a grounding oil and was used throughout history for connecting to God and having your mind in a spiritual space.

Remember our affirmations and why they are so important? As we dive into growth, affirmations like, "I am safe," "I am at peace," "I am loved", or even simply, "I trust" may help you remind yourself of the truth. When we have experienced PTSD, and are striving for growth, reminding ourselves of what is truth is critical. Triggers are rooted in experiences, not truth. Triggers come when a situation reminds us of an experience again; it's not what is true of what is happening at that moment.

Combined with inhaling essential oils, these affirmations will create new brain pathways. "I learn from all of life's experiences" is another beautiful affirmation that will propel you forward. Hear me, if your story involves abuse, this does not excuse the behavior of the person who has abused you. What it does do is help you find space to forgive, and move forward, to a life of healing and pouring out onto others who have experienced a similar trauma. Not forgiving is like drinking poison and expecting someone else to die. It's just not going to happen. Unforgiveness keeps us stuck and trapped in negativity. Forgiveness sets us free.

Learning from life's experiences is what makes us the amazing people God created us to be. As scripture reminds us, "what the enemy meant for evil and harm, God will use it for GOOD." Neuroplasticity is the ability of the brain to form and reorganize synaptic connections. Simply put- our brains can physically change. Just twenty short years ago neuroscientist would have believed that someone with a traumatic brain injury was just doomed to suffer with brain damage, never to recover from it. Today we know now it's simply not true. Our brains can heal and change.

In addition to this information on emotional releasing and healing, epigenetics is something to be well versed in. We'll keep this simple as you can easily do a quick Google search on epigenetics. Epigenetics is the study of changes in organisms caused by modification of gene expression rather than alteration of the genetic code itself. In other words, our genetic code contains all we are, and can be. Studying the entirety of that that is the study of genetics in general. Epigenetics is the study of how some genes are expressed while others are not. There are four key things you need to know about epigenetics.

1. Epigenetics control genes.
2. Epigenetics is everywhere.
3. Epigenetics makes us unique.
4. Epigenetic changes are reversible. That's my personal favorite.

We received the diagnosis of malignant melanoma for our son, with a bonus of "hey guess what mom and dad! Your other children have a 50% higher chance of getting this cancer too!" Oh hell no. Not only was I determined to cure my son forever of this, I was determined to keep that killer out of my other children.

Our genes are controlled by this through two things, nature and nurture. Nature being what determines a cell's specialization (e.g., skin cell, blood cell, hair cell, liver cells, etc.) as a baby develops into a bigger baby through gene expression (active) or silencing (dormant). And nurture being environmental stimuli that can also cause genes to be turned off or turned on. What's in our environment? Stress, toxin overload, poor diet? Speaking of food, like I said, epigenetic impacts are everywhere! From what you eat to where you live, to who you interact with, when you sleep, and how you exercise, all of these can eventually cause chemical modifications around the genes that will turn those genes on or off over time.

Everyone wants to be individual and epigenetics proves that we are just that, unique in every way. Think of it, why do some of us have blonde hair or darker skin? Why do some of us love the taste of mushrooms or beets? Why are some of us more out going than others? The different combinations of genes that are turned on or off are what make each one of us unique. It bares repeating that this is my favorite; epigenetic changes are reversible. In other words, a gene that has been turned on can be turned off. With 20,000+ genes, what will be the result of the different combinations of genes being turned on or off? The possible arrangements are tremendous! Let's say we could map every single cause and effect of the different combinations, and if we could reverse the gene's state to keep the good while eliminating the bad, then we could quite possibly cure cancer, slow aging, stop obesity, and so much more. For now, I share these things with you so that you understand at a minimum that your story can change. Your brain can change. How you are now may not be truly who you are. Your body condition, though "hereditary", can absolutely be reversed. Your body may have switched on a genetic malfunction all because of one event, one trauma.

As we discussed with neuroplasticity, our brains can physically change. This is amazing news given the fact that many PTSD sufferers have some form of brain alteration. This will absolutely transform your mental state and growth as you learn and then apply this info specifically to your brain. In studies performed at Vienna and Berlin Universities, researchers discovered that sesquiterpenes in the essential oils of Cedar wood, Sandalwood and Frankincense, can increase levels of oxygen in the brain by up to 28 percent. By the way, these can be found in an essential oil blend called Brain Power, a blend specifically formulated to help mental recovery.

Using these oils often, 3-4 times a day, can really start to repair damage that's occurred in the brain. For emotional trauma, these oils can help release fear and worry with peace of mind. Also, the oils help the mind release the negative or traumatic memories and hold on to positive memories.

We have talked a lot about journaling and affirmations and prayer. These are perfect additions as we heal mentally and spiritually. We must not neglect the physical part of healing our brain. Essential oils will allow the brain to speak to the cells and create healing within the cells. In addition, our cells need food so we can strengthen our bodies. Taking supplements is an excellent way to feed our cells while we heal.

If there is brain damage- below are two supplements that are amazing to repair and feed the brain. Think of it this way; like our body, if our brain is not getting the food it needs, it cannot heal properly.

MindWise is a supplement with a high proportion of unsaturated fatty acids and omega-3 fatty acids which are critical for brain health and function, specifically after trauma. Fat is brain food. It also contains bioidentical COQ10, Vitamin D3, and other beneficial ingredients to the brain.

Ningxia Nitro is a cognitive fitness beverage that includes D-Ribose, green tea extract, mulberry leaf extract, Korean ginseng extract, choline and essential oils that may assist the body's inflammatory response to irritation and injury – crucial after traumatic brain incidents.

May I encourage you in this, be gentle on your brain as it recovers, take your brain supplements and apply your brain oils consistently each day, with intention.

Post Traumatic Growth also includes Emotional Recovery. I know, I know, kinda obvious right? Yet we tend to lump all the recovery into one group, forgetting that emotional is different from spiritual is different from mental. They are different ways to heal.

So after trauma, some people's social cues change. This is an aspect of how we can grow. Whether someone is triggered because of a type of relationship or because of uncontrolled stress responses; feelings of anxiousness or frustration; or a mental block against certain activities, recognizing the triggers and responding appropriately will create the GROWTH we are looking for emotionally.

Chapter 11

Growth from Trauma - Steps

To participate in the growth from trauma steps, you'll want to have your essential oils handy. Valor, Inner Child, Forgiveness, Joy, Cedar Wood, Sacred Mountain and Trauma Life. Valor should be used prior to social events, group events, or new interactions post-trauma, this oil blend will help build your confidence. Also- a great oil for introverts. This oil can go a long way toward heading off triggers.

Joy should be applied over your heart using this affirmation: "I am blessed with healthy relationships." or "I am at peace and full of joy in all situations".

There is a protocol that you could walk through, in which may be a huge benefit to you or your children. We have walked each of our children through this at various times throughout the months and years, and can I tell you, it makes a HUGE difference in their attitudes toward one another.

side note this is a perfect way to deal with issues that you are fully aware of and have no clue how to remove the sting of the memory.

Step 1:
Inner Child: The greatest power that a person can have is to know "who they are," and this is often

disconnected due to trauma. This blend helps connect you with your identity. Simply inhale & place a drop on the thumb and touch the roof of your mouth to stimulate the pituitary/pineal gland, saying the affirmation "I am enough."

Step 2:
Forgiveness: Can't sleep due to rage, anger, hatred, nightmares? This blend helps to release hurtful memories and move beyond emotional barriers. Rub around the navel, inhale and rub on wrists. Repeat "I choose to forgive".

Step 3:
Trauma Life: A powerful blend to help release buried emotional trauma resulting from accidents, neglect, abuse, assault, memories and more. Inhale several times & apply over liver. Allow memories to surface, do not push them back. If tears or heavy emotions rise up, remind yourself, feelings are like waves, they will not last forever, ride it out and release them.

Step 4:
Repeat Inner Child, only this time, picture a positive memory. As you breathe in Inner Child picture that memory, seal it in with the oil.

Step 5:
Take an oil that represents strength, perhaps Cedar wood or Sacred Mountain. Apply 3 drops to your

palms and breathe in. As you do, visualize something that you see as having unending strength. Hold that image in your mind as you breathe in the oil. You might take this time to ground yourself as you visualize, creating a feeling of strength in you.

Chapter 12

Brain Dump

For this next chapter, have your journal or spare paper and pen, and your 'brain essential oils' ie- Cedar wood, Brainpower, Clarity and/or Envision. You'll want to have Release handy, especially after I walk you through the brain dump.

What exactly is a Brain Dump? So glad you asked! Sometimes our brain is a mess, cluttered with thoughts that do not serve us or the purpose for which we were created. In this situation, a brain dump is a must. It's when you take every single thought you currently are thinking and dump it on paper. You do not care about penmanship, or spelling. You just write, and write fast. Exhaust yourself as you write, do not think of anything but what flows from your brain, out of the pen and onto the paper.

When we were walking through a particularly rough season, our family started a habit of brain dumping before we got moving with our day. It helped with grumpy attitudes and harder hearts before we started the school day. For children, you can make this a totally safe space to write what is really going on in their minds. They may typically want to say only what they think we want to hear, so if they're allowed to dump whatever is on their mind, no judgment, no mom or dad or siblings reading it later, they will get it out on paper.

The beauty of this exercise is we are able to look at it objectively. We can look at what we wrote and ask ourselves, is it true? Is it helpful? Does it serve us? What a beautiful way to teach children to capture their thoughts and recognize the thoughts for what they are.

First thing in the morning, maybe after teeth brushing, simply take 5 minutes and wrote whatever was on your mind.

~it's cold out
~I feel tired
~why am I up early
and so on.

What happens when we let those thoughts ruminate in our brains is we may become anxious, stressed or so frustrated that we can't focus. Worse yet, we let these thoughts cloud our day, when in reality, there is no truth in them. They have zero bearing on what is happening. What if there is truth in the thoughts? What if what you are ruminating about is something truly terrible going on in your life? Diagnosis, marriage crisis, wayward child, financial pressures weighing you down? There is no better time than this to brain dump! Get that noise out on paper so you can take every thought captive and make it obedient to Christ. That's all you are doing, taking the negative thoughts and saying, "hey, Jesus, take this, I don't want it." Guess what, He gladly takes it. He takes it and throws it far away. He will take them and then remind you that you already have, through the power of the Holy Spirit, love, joy, peace, patience, goodness, kindness, gentleness, faithfulness and self control. You already possess the things you need to think clearly, to dwell on the lovely, the admirable, the excellent. Just because something is true, doesn't make it positive. Nothing good ever comes from worrying about a bad situation. Instead, pray, be thankful, have faith that your God will never leave you or forsake you. Have faith in His word and His promises. Claim those promises for yourself, over you and your situation.

"We are destroying speculations and every lofty thing raised up against the knowledge of God, and we are taking every thought captive to the obedience of Christ." 2 Corinthians 10:5

Look at your brain dump again. Take a long look at what you wrote.

- Is there truth?
- How much of what you wrote were comments of frustration?
- How much of your notes were positive and full of joy?

Now, write a new thought surrounding what you just wrote, only this time flip it. Right it in the positive form. i.e., "it's early and I feel tired, but praise God for life today!"

"There's this issues, but I am so filled with joy today, none of that matters".

"This is going on but I know Who sits on the throne of Heaven and He is always in control."

While you do this, get creative, use colors, write all over the page, write it backwards if you have to. When we go about things differently, our brain will WAKE UP! Some of us need to get WOKE in order to see truth as they could be. Do things in a different way so that it shakes up the nonsense that might be in our minds, so that we can see things as they are. Most importantly, make sure the truth sticks. Notice too as you make this a daily practice, you will start to flip your thoughts automatically. When stuck in traffic, you'll remind yourself what a blessing it is to be able to listen a little longer to that audible book or the worship music. When your children are fighting or acting like fools, you'll find yourself thanking God you have them, and that they are passionate, outspoken people.

Be mindful of your thoughts, in all situations today and everyday, especially the more pesky ones. Note how you respond, what your thoughts are. Choose to respond in the best way, a way that shows who you truly want to be.

Chapter 13

Rewrite The Story

Write your new story, the story you desire to be true of your day. This is the best part of brain detoxing. Much like body detoxing, once the toxins are flushed out, you replace it with healthy nutrients. In brain detoxing, we must now replace the toxic thoughts with something life giving, creating a habit of positivity rather than revert back to our old ways. This is how we take the trainings, workshops and seminars we sit through and make them our reality. We step by step replace the old with the new.

Ultimately, this is a perfect practice for writing the story you are creating for your life. Everything you want also wants you. You must take action to achieve it. Today that action looks like writing a story. As you are writing, remember that we have the ability to use our marvelous imagination. It's one of the things that separates us from animals, we can think, reason, imagine. Imagine big, imagine different, let your imagination go wild!

If you could create a new story for yourself, what would it look like? Would you be looking around at the faces of the people who have chosen to walk with you to freedom of health? How would you describe that? What would it be like to watch them take ownership and change their lives alongside you? In your new story, are you feeling alive, invigorated and FREE?

What steps can you take each day to start getting an actual visual of what your new story looks like? Do you run? Could you take that run and picture yourself running with others doing the same thing you are doing? Are you involved in your community somehow? What would it look like to have your community forever changed because you are? Ask the question, "How can I?" This simple question keeps dreams directly before you and will keep from thinking of why it's not possible. Your brain will automatically search for the answer.

How do we connect several of our senses as we recreate and think and pray? Using our essential oils, drawing out colorful pictures, listening to powerful life giving music as we become creative in the process. Choose an essential oil as you work through this step that you most connect with. The oil that if it were possible, you would swim in it as an ocean of oil. Which is that for you? Is it Magnify Your Purpose? Perhaps Grounding? Even Into The Future so you can get a crystal clear picture firmly in your mind. Once you have your story written, place it where you will see it often throughout the day. Read it as much as possible.

Conclusion

Have you now completed the steps described in this book, or maybe you're about to? If so, there are some things you should know.

Deciding is one step, actually walking in freedom, of grabbing what you are believing for, is a whole other ball game.
Something that hinders some folks from taking this final step in brain detox is called negative positive reinforcement.

This looks like hanging on to old feelings and paradigms because when you share them with others, they may sympathize or even empathize with you. It's a positive response to a negative pattern. When someone gives you pity because of all you've gone through, the body releases a feel good hormone, which, well, feels good. This pattern may keep some from truly walking it out.

Standing strong and grounded and believing for the life you desire doesn't always bring praise from others. In fact, it can bring the opposite. After all, your circles may enjoy how at one point, you felt angst more than you felt joy. Misery loves company. Like attracts like. Now that you are creating freedom in your life, be aware of your patterns of old creeping in.

Action steps:

As I mentioned in the beginning, read this book three times. I hope you did not start the work before you finished reading this through.

If you're like me, you totally blew off my suggestion, got a chapter or two into it and said, "nah, I can do this without reading three times! I mean, it's not that difficult." Except, I have a suspicion you may have had a couple of blocks along the way. You see, this course was designed as a college level class, to take and pour into and receive a new level of understanding and awareness each time you complete it.

So let's do this again. You have now completed this book. Go back to the beginning, perhaps with a new journal and a fresh batch of essential oils.
Allow yourself to gain a deeper bit of wisdom and work through the steps, slowly. Thoughtfully.

Finally, if this is your third time passing through, I pray it has sunk so deep into your soul that you are compelled to take what you have learned and now you are sharing it. I am a huge believer in keeping information in circulation. Don't close this book and just move along. Share the idea with someone, or a group of people.